13 Keys to Wellness Success

Ashley & Ashley

DEDICATION

To all those embarking on a positive lifestyle may you continue to flourish each and every day.

CONTENTS

ACKNOWLEDGMENTS

Though your journey may not be easy, anything worth having is worth fighting for. Keep pushing.

1. BE PATIENT

You must set realistic and attainable goals for yourself. You will not lose two pants size in a day nor will you lose fifty pounds safely in a month. Be patient your desired change will come.

You may have heard the phrase "Patience is a virtue" at some point in your life. It is a term widely used with minimal understanding. Patience is not just sitting and waiting for something to happen. Patience is truly a combination of your ability and your capacity to accept, tolerate and endure unfavorable delays without getting frustrated, upset or wavering in motivation and determination.

To practice patience, you must be actively engaging and preforming. If you are not engaging and pursuing a goal then you do not allow yourself to exhibit patience. Allow yourself the opportunity and privilege of activating and utilizing your patience. Patience can be ignited in an abundance of circumstances. To be patient requires effort and consistency. Patience is a true virtue because it is far and few between.

TIPS

- Be mindful

- Live in the moment

- Think before you speak or act

- Take your time

- Shift your perspective

YOUR THOUGHTS:

_____

_____

_____

_____

_____

_____

_____

_____

_____

_____

_____

_____

_____

_____

_____

_____

_____

_____

_____

_____

_____

_____

_____

_____

_____

_____

2. COMMIT YOURSELF

Embarking on a new journey can be fun and exciting. It can also be intimidating and challenging. When you feel tempted to reassess your commitment indefinitely…also known as quitting… reframe from doing so. Give it some time and STICK WITH IT!

Commitment is scary because change is scary. To be able to commit you must be able to accept change. People often fear change and commitment because they go hand in hand. To commit means you take on this certain level of dedication, devotion, and loyalty. Think of your wellness commitment as a dedication to yourself. This commitment is your amount of loyalty to yourself and no one else. If you cannot commit to yourself than who can you truly commit to?

Commitment should not feel like a liability. Every day we commit ourselves to someone or something. We commit to school, work, family, friends, etc. but we somehow manage to not make or simply break commitments we make to ourselves. Let this be the turning point to that cycle and COMMIT! Commit to personal wellness, health, happiness and most importantly commit to yourself. You absolutely, 100% deserve it and are beyond worth it. Allow yourself to be healthy and commit to yourself so that you are able to maintain your other commitments in a healthy manner.

TIPS

- Be genuinely committed to yourself

- Consider your feelings

- Avoid self-deprecating comments

- Gain clarity

- Utilize self-discipline

- Invest in yourself

YOUR THOUGHTS:

_____

_____

_____

_____

_____

_____

_____

_____

_____

_____

_____

_____

_____

_____

_____

_____

_____

_____

_____

_____

_____

_____

_____

_____

_____

3. WORKOUT

Get moving! Any exercise is better than no exercise at all. 10 minutes a day can make a world of difference for your body and your efforts. No matter the type of exercise, extent or intensity of the activity do it!

Working out is not something that comes easy to everyone. My-oh-my what a true privilege it is to do so. Working out is something that so many people take for granted and do not realize. When you change your perception of working out you are able to see that some humans are literally groaning and moaning about being able to walk at a brisk pace, to bend and twist, to move their legs…their bodies. How ungrateful we must be to gripe about mobility.

Working out is such a powerful tool. Working out exercises both your mind and body, it is a two for one activity. Your mental health is equally as important as your physical wellbeing and working out engages both your physical and mental state of being. Start small if you have to by simply walking further distances than from the refrigerator to the couch. Go for a walk around the neighborhood. Build on that and walk around the neighborhood twice. Commit, be patient and workout.

Develop your physical fitness level at your pace. Set mini workout milestones and achieve them. You are able . Remember that working out may seem like a task to some but what a joy it is to those that are not physical able. Start with a small workout and increase it as you naturally get stronger both physically and mentally.

TIPS

- Make wellness a habit

- Work one muscle group at a time

- Finish every exercise

- Be consistent

- Water is your best friend

- Remember why you started

- Ask yourself if you will regret not working out

- Compete with yourself

- You can do this

YOUR THOUGHTS:

_____

_____

_____

_____

_____

_____

_____

_____

_____

_____

_____

_____

_____

_____

_____

_____

_____

_____

_____

_____

_____

_____

_____

_____

_____

_____

4. EAT CLEAN

Eating clean is a big part of the challenge. Being able to conquer this feat is amazing in itself and it can eliminate a lot of the "guilt" some people may feel when they embark on a new lifestyle journey. A lot of positive change can be accomplished when you eat clean. Fuel your body with what it needs and desires. Begin to feel better from the inside out.

Meal time is a big player on your journey to wellness success. Food is a central part of society, it is used to meet basic needs, celebrate, mourn and cope and cannot simply be avoided. Changing your eating habits is one of the first things you should do as you embark on this journey. It is a great way to start your journey and the impact of simply changing your eating habits will astound you.

Does this mean you must sacrifice flavor or taste? Absolutely not! You just have to sacrifice unnecessary fats, sugars and bad cholesterol that breed negativity to your body. There are plenty of foods that you can eat that taste great and are great for your body. Food must be mastered.

<u>TIPS</u>

- Do not skip breakfast or any meals

- Drink water!

- Vegetables are your friend

- Proteins are to be eaten

- Minimize your sugar intake

- PORTION control! Bigger is not better and you do not need "more"

- Snacks are great!

- Eat fiber rich foods

- Prepare your healthy meals

- Easy on the sodium intake

YOUR THOUGHTS:

_____

_____

_____

_____

_____

_____

_____

_____

_____

_____

_____

_____

_____

5. GUARD YOUR MINDSET

The mind is a powerful, powerful, powerful thing. Preparing your mind is essential for your success. Disengage from those whom pose a threat to your success. The mental aspect is just as important as the physical aspect of the journey.

Once you have made your mind up to achieve wellness do not let anyone or anything detour you. The mental aspect is half the journey and the challenge. Thoughts and words can build you , mold you and impact your life and behaviors continuously. What you believe is essential to your success.

Daily affirmations are a great tool to have in your arsenal for moments when you start to have doubts or your mindset waivers. Your mind is in control of your entire body. Why would you not protect and guard it? The only limits you have are those you place on yourself.

AFFIRMATIONS

- I can achieve greatness.

- I love and accept myself.

- I will do my best at all times with all things.

- My body is healthy, my mind is intelligent and my soul is peaceful.

- I can do anything.

- I can only affect what I contribute to.

- I must build a foundation for my life and choose its contents wisely.

- My potential is limitless

YOUR THOUGHTS:

_____

_____

_____

_____

_____

_____

_____

_____

_____

_____

_____

_____

_____

_____

_____

_____

_____

_____

_____

_____

_____

_____

_____

_____

_____

_____

_____

6. <u>STAY</u> POSITIVE

Keeping a positive mind frame will be mandatory to your journey. You will need to be positive when you start your journey and continue to be just as positive if not even more so as the days pass and it seems to be more challenging for you. Any negative change in your mindset can negatively impact your journey.

Your amount of positivity can either make you or break you along this journey. If you can stay positive and speak life unto yourself and your journey, then you can truly fuel and propel yourself into unexplored revelations and circumstances. Keep your spirits high. The more positivity you have and utilize the further you will go.

Your positivity will also affect how you perceive your wellness journey to be. If you think it is miserable then it will be miserable. Negativity only breads negativity. Change your mindset think about all the positive emotional and physical benefits and this can be one of the greatest and rewarding journey of your life.

TIPS

- Do not let your fears hold you back

- Find the silver lining in all negative situations

- Make your environment positive. Your environment is a major factor.

- Do not make a mountain out of a molehill

- Be gracious

- Believe you will succeed

YOUR THOUGHTS:

_____

_____

_____

_____

_____

_____

_____

_____

_____

_____

_____

_____

_____

_____

_____

_____

_____

_____

_____

_____

_____

_____

_____

_____

_____

_____

_____

7. SAY "YES!"

It is so easy to self-sabotage your positive lifestyle change. Giving in to temptation too often can be detrimental to your success. Do not contemplate making good decisions to workout, eat clean and be positive. Say "Yes!" to any kind of movement, say "Yes!" to eating clean, Say "Yes!" to positive thoughts and compliments.

It can be so easy and comfortable to second guess the necessary things needed to positively change your wellness. Old habits can be hard to break but it is not called a challenge for nothing.

Going into your wellness journey you should be fully aware that it will require you to say and do things that you have not been doing as frequently as you should have been. You will be forced to step out of your comfort zone, elevate your mental and physical wellbeing, push yourself, grow and expand. In order for you to accomplish these thing you will absolutely positively have to say "yes". Think about any successful person in the world. Do you think that they said "No" or "I cannot" very often when they were trying to achieve their goal? No, they did not and you should not either. Embrace the journey and the change ahead. Say "YES"!

TIPS

- Say yes to change

- Say yes to yourself

- Say yes to new foods

- Say yes to movement

- Say yes to positivity

- Say yes to new people in new places such as the gym or market

- Say yes to your body

- Say yes to water

- Say yes to each nutritious meal

- Say yes to heart health

- Say yes to strong muscles

- Say yes to challenges

- Say yes to exercise

- Say yes to vegetables

- Say yes to fruits

- Say yes to new beginnings

YOUR THOUGHTS:

_____

_____

_____

_____

_____

_____

_____

_____

_____

_____

_____

_____

_____

_____

_____

_____

_____

_____

_____

_____

_____

_____

_____

_____

_____

_____

8. DISCIPLINE

This key goes hand in hand with the say "Yes!" Key. Have some self-discipline throughout this journey. Be disciplined to the goal(s) you've set for yourself and for your health. Be disciplined when it comes to eating clean. Be disciplined when it comes to being active and accomplishing daily activities. Be disciplined when it comes to disengaging in negative counterproductive thoughts and behaviors.

Discipline is one of my absolute favorite keys because it is such a personal key that cannot be influenced by anyone else but yourself. It is such a personal attribute that truly speaks for itself. You have got to have some self-discipline in your life. Self-discipline can and should be used in every area of your life. If you do not have any self-discipline, then you will set yourself up for self-sabotage and disappointment every single time. Anything that you do in life will require some lever of self-discipline. The more you have the better off you will be. If you do not have any I strongly recommend you gain some to avoid a vicious cycle of disappointment.

TIPS

- Remove temptations

- Eat regularly and healthily

- Continue moving forward

- Practice self-forgiveness

- Reward yourself for accomplishments

- Control your habit. 40% of behavior is habit-driven

YOUR THOUGHTS:

_____

_____

_____

_____

_____

_____

_____

_____

_____

_____

_____

_____

_____

_____

_____

_____

_____

_____

_____

_____

_____

_____

_____

_____

_____

_____

9. CONSISTENCY

Consistency promotes change which leads to success. Being consistent is essential. Don't allow yourself to be inconsistent too often. It is counterproductive to your journey and success. Poor consistency leads to stagnation. Be consistent in working out, be consistent in how you choose to fuel your body and be consistent in your positive mindset!

Be consistent in every area of your life. Without consistency there will be no progression. A lack of consistency results in a mindless endless circle of running on a hamster wheel. Set a goal, plan ahead and execute. Do not give up when things get challenging. Try, try and try harder. Each and every challenge or barrier will mold you to be stronger. Think of hard times as a learning experience instead of an optical. Do

not be easily deterred. Consistency is key at all time.

TIPS

- Have a routine

- Do things you need to do even if you do not feel like
  it

- Take responsibility

- Focus on the process

- Change your thinking

- Build your willpower

- Do not think negatively

YOUR THOUGHTS:

_____

_____

_____

_____

_____

_____

_____

_____

_____

_____

_____

_____

10. DRIVE

Never give up! Rome wasn't built in a day and your total transformation won't be either. Make sure you motivate you. Do not leave your success in someone else hands. If your drive is slacking, then your results will surely suffer.

This key depends solely on you and you cannot depend on anyone else to fuel your drive. Anything worth having is worth fighting for and anything worth doing is worth doing well. This process is really and truly a lifestyle choice. Once you reach your desired goal you will have to work daily to maintain it.

Do not adjust your goals to match your drive but rather adjust your drive to match your goals. You can do it; you will make it.

TIPS

- Avoid negative people

- Build your support group

- Create a vision for your life

- Unclutter your mental and physical space

- Practice self-care

- Prioritize

- Celebrate your achievements

- Take action

- Impress yourself first and foremost

- Play to your strengths

YOUR THOUGHTS:

_____

_____

_____

_____

_____

_____

_____

_____

_____

_____

_____

_____

_____

11. PLAN AHEAD

Better prepared than sorry! Allow yourself to have a smoother day and be less tempted to stray away from your goals by being prepared. You can achieve this by pre planning your meals & snacks, food prepping & scheduling your weekly activities in advance.

Having a plan will make this journey smoother for all those involved. Would you jump in deep murky water without look or having some type of plan of action? I do not think so. At best you know your motivation for jumping. Before you beginning this journey and all throughout this journey know your motivation, your drive. After you have your motivation only then can you be able to plan ahead.

TIPS

- Know what you are preparing for

- Adjust when needed

- Be honest with yourself

- Keep your long term goal in mind

- Maintain momentum

- Allow flexibility

YOUR THOUGHTS:

_____

_____

_____

_____

_____

_____

12. SET A GOAL

What are you working towards? What is your motivation? Set a goal that is realistic and obtainable and work towards it every minute of every day of every week until it is reached. One you accomplish your goal, set a new goal and go for it! Continue to grow & achieve positive lifestyle changes!

What are you working towards? Once you figure it out write it down. Goals are forever changing and evolving as you grow and develop. Reaching your goal and being able and set a new goal is such an accomplishment and you should be extremely proud when you reach each and every goal.

Goals provide you with vision and purpose and short term motivation. It is an excellent idea to set short term goals and long term goals related to your physical, mental and emotional wellbeing.

TIPS

- Decide your small term goals

- Decide your long term goals

- Write all your goals down

- Set realistic goals

- Break your goals down and plan your first step

- Never give up

- Celebrate each goal accomplishment no matter how minute they may seem to you

- Make your goals attainable

- Set measurable goals

YOUR THOUGHTS:

_____

_____

_____

_____

_____

_____

_____

_____

_____

_____

_____

_____

13. THRIVE

Make it happen! You must decide, believe, & actively seek in order to achieve!

Your success is not comparable to anyone else's success and you should never compare the two. *Your* success, *your* drive, *your* goals, *your* plans, *your* consistency, *your* commitment, *your* patience and *your* behaviors are just that. **Yours** and **yours** alone. The only common denominator in the equation is *you.*

Your level of success is up to you and it is very important to remember that. You can do absolutely anything that you set your mind to and work hard for. Do not let anyone or anything be a determining factor. You must rise above and overcome any and all obstacle. All the needed tools are at your fingertips. It is up to you to live your best life. It is up to you to be fruitful. The decision is 100% in your more than capable hands. You must choose to *THRIVE!*

TIPS

- Be kind to yourself

- Utilize positive thinking

- Be your greatest fan

- Be actively involved in life

- Eliminate what does not elevate your fullest potential

- Eat real food

- Cultivate relationships

- Be insightful

- Get to know yourself

- Nourishment over stimulates

- Live in the present

- Trust yourself

YOUR THOUGHTS:

_____

_____

_____

_____

_____

_____

_____

_____

_____

_____

_____

_____

_____

_____

_____

_____

_____

_____

_____

_____

_____

_____

GOALS & ASPIRATIONS TOWARDS POSITVE CHANGES...

1. _____

   _____

   _____

   _____

2. _____

   _____

   _____

   _____

3. _____

   _____

   _____

   _____

4. _____

_____

_____

_____

5. _____

_____

_____

_____

6. _____

_____

_____

_____

7. _____

_____

_____

_____

8. _____

_____

_____

_____

9. _____

_____

_____

_____

10. _____

_____

_____

_____

_____

_____

_____

_____

_____

_____

_____

_____

_____

I AM GRATFUL FOR......

1. _____

_____

_____

_____

_____

2. _____

_____

_____

_____

3. _____

_____

_____

_____

_____

_____

4. _____

_____

_____

_____

_____

_____

5. _____

_____

_____

_____

_____

_____

JOURNAL

_____

_____

_____

_____

_____

_____

_____

_____

_____

_____

_____

ABOUT THE AUTHOR

Ashley & Ashley live in Texas. They are strong believers and advocates for strength perspectives. They believe that anything is possible by faith and hard work. They are the authors of many other books to include cook books and children's books. For more information, products and services visit their website CIRC by Ashley & Ashley at www.circtoday.com